I0758875

ACID REFLUX & HEARTBURN DIET PLAN

Detailed Guide in Preventing, Treating and Healing Your Heartburn by Taking Diets That Is Free Of Gluten and Acidic Content, Better Living Habit and No Use of Drugs

BY:

Doctor Eliza Parker

Copyright@2020

Table of Content

CHAPTER ONE

DESCRIBING LOW ACID FOOD THAT IS GOOD FOR YOUR REFLUX DIET

Research has made us to know that food that is high in acidic content leads to heartburn. Practicing food low in acidic content is not difficult as you are thinking.

Your present state of obesity can be a concern for you at the moment but sooner it will be a forgotten issue with simple application of intermittent fasting.

Person who is suffering from regular heartburn will now how important it is to avoid any thing that causes heartburn. Food that has high volume of saturated fat can help weaken the pressure of the sphincter muscle that resides at the top of the stomach. If the sphincter muscle is not tightly shut, it will allow the stomach acid and food backwash to the esophagus and throats thereby create heartburn.

One simple way to avoid heartburn is to keep acid separately from mixing up with the food we eat. Avoiding acidic food, keep acid content far from the stomach.

Going back to chemistry, water has a PH value of 7 which is sometimes called neutral. Any value lower than 7 is acidic value while value higher than 7 is refers to as alkaline. Note that a drop in 1 value of the PH scale means 10 times its acidic level. This shows that a small drop in acidic scale indicates a high level of acidic content in your diet. The acceptable acid value of stomach PH is between 1 and 4. The PH value for the stomach is low due to the gastric acids it secretes for the breaking down of food.'' Explain by Michelle Duong Davenport, MA, and Researcher at NYU School of Medicine.

Expert discourages us from eating some types of food and beverages such as peppermint, caffeine, chocolate and alcohol especially persons suffering from reflux so as to prevent heartburn.

Research also shows that 20 persons were treated with proton pump inhibitor (PPI) and H2 blocker and still suffers reflux symptoms but gets better improvement with regular intake of low acidic diets for two weeks.

More researches are needed to know what low acidic content in our diets can be of help to the body. Other health benefits of eating low acidic diets are listed below;

- ✓ Decrease the rate of tooth decay

✓ Lower risk of fracture of the bone

It is advice to tell your doctor before taking the low acidic diets so as to guide you if you are having any health related issues. Here are the right low acid diets listed below;

- BANANA

Banana is known for alkalinity content and not acidity. It is rich in vitamin B, fiber and the building up of potassium that works well for bones and the heart. Taking banana in it raw state is simply the best source of nutrient. Banana can be taking anytime in form of snacks or in between meal. Banana can be mash and taking as substitute for fat.

- A SKINLESS CHICKEN

Skinless chicken is considered as another diet that is low in acid content but has a high level of protein. An intake of 4 ounce portion of skinless chicken will provide you with two-thirds of your required daily nutrient. When you fry the skinless chicken in greasy oil, it tends to trigger heartburn. Try and prepare the chicken with ingredient that will not cause heartburn. Use spices that will less trigger your reflux.

- APPLE

Apple is another source of low acid diet that is high in fiber. An intake of fiber will make you stay full for a longer time thereby reducing rate at which you eat during the day time. Preventing an increase in blood sugar and the lowering of cholesterol is possible with an intake of apple. The skin of apple fruit contains polyphenols and flavonoids which is also good for you.

- FISH

Almost all diet adds fish to it for more nutrients. This is an excellent source of protein which is presented in low acid diets. A fish called salmon is rich in omega-3 fatty acids which plays vital role in the eyes, heart and joint. Fish may also prevent cancer diseases for some person suffering from this ailment. Avoid adding seasonings to fish which might tend to cause heartburn to human being.

- OATMEAL

Oatmeal is recommended as a breakfast meal for persons who desire a low-acid diet. Oatmeal is high in fiber and it helps in building cardiovascular health and balances the blood sugar level.

When taking a hot bowl of oatmeal in addition with fruits, make sure you avoid the fruit that is high in acidic content. Fruits high in acid contents are strawberries, cranberries and blueberries.

- ALMONDS

Almond is refers to as alkaline in nature when compare to other nuts that are acidic such as; pecans, walnuts and cashew. Almond nut contains monounsaturated fatty acid and omega-3 fatty acids for the protection of the heart while the high fiber it contains helps to keep you full always during the day.

It is advice to use almond nut in place of other nut due to its low acidic content. It also contains Vitamin E which is known as a natural antioxidant.

- WHOLE GRAIN BROWN RICE

Whether you are following low acid diet or not, brown rice is known as a healthy choice food that is richly high in fiber. The fiber does digestive tract regulation, boost healthy heart and vitamin B abundance which help to maintain body energy.

- MELON

All melon is accepted as meal. Such melon is watermelon, honeydew and cantaloupe.

- POTATOES

All root vegetables are good source of food.

- EGG WHITE

The egg white is a rich source of protein and has low acid content. Don't eat the yolk since it tends to cause other symptoms.

- GREEN VEGGIES

Example of green veggies that has low acid content is Broccoli, green beans, cauliflower, asparagus, and celery.

Merely looking at a food will not automatically tells you the acidic content it posses. Get the name of the food and search for it PH value so as to know how acidic it is. The lower the PH value the higher the acidic content.

PH value for lemon juice is 2.0 and it is more acidic than a food having a PH value of 5.0. other low- acid cook book might list recommended food that are of low acid content.

ADDITIONAL FOOD THAT CAN RELIEF HEARTBURN

Important herbs and food that is use to treat upset stomach and reflux. It might not work for everyone.

- ✓ FENNEL

This is refer to as a crunchy vegetable which has a licorice flavor and act as an addition to salads. There are tendency that fennel can improve digestion. It has a low acidic value of 6.9.

✓ GINGER

This is a good natural herb that treats upset stomach. It is inactive when it comes to reflux.

✓ PARSLEY

It is seen that the sprig of parsley that you are holding is not for decoration rather it is use traditionally for the treatment of upset stomach for many years. Parsley also poses some acid reflux.

NOTE: eating the right diet will really assist greatly in fighting your heartburn. No matter how rich your food may look like, trigger content in the food will still cause reflux. A little quantity of ginger in your food can cause heartburn.

CHAPTER TWO

THE SIMPLIFY ALKALINE DIETS THAT YOU CAN OR CAN NOT TAKE

The different food we eat has different PH value which might be less or more acidic. Below is the alkaline list of food needed so as to stay clear from neutral and acidic food.

ACIDIC FOODS

- Fish
- Poultry
- Meat
- Alcohol
- Dairy
- Peanuts and walnuts
- Eggs
- Grains

NEUTRAL FOODS
- Sugar
- Natural fats
- Starches

ALKALINE FOODS

- Legumes
- Fruits
- vegetables

No special meal plan is given to direct you on what to eat as alkaline food but rather you are to develop the best meal plan for yourself. You can search further for a correct diet meal plan online or from a trusted diet cookbooks shop.

SCIENCE PERSPECTIVE ABOUT FOOD AND PH

The PH level of your body varies from one part to the other and it is higher when compare to the PH value of the food you eat. The stomach has a high acidic content for digestion likewise the skin and the woman vaginal. The vaginal acidic contents, guide the body from harmful bacteria.

Your body PH value is mainly regulated and maintain by the lungs and kidney. The PH value of human blood ranges from 7.2 to 7.45.

Persons having challenges with malfunctioning of the lungs and kidney should see medical personnel for help. A ventilator or dialysis should be given to such patients so as to get a balance PH level.

Your body PH level cannot be change by the amount of food you eat

CAN EATING ALKALINE DIET CAUSE WEIGHT LOSS

Most persons claim that eating alkaline diet will tend to reduce body weight but such claim are not true. Alkaline diets are mainly eating for the prevention and treatment of diseases. Chronic conditions and diseases such as cancer and kidney ailment may be treated from daily intake of alkaline diets..

If you follow a well plan Mediterranean diet, it may tend to reduce the risk of cancer in human being.

EAT WELL TO GET A HEALTHY HEART

It is also research with better findings that the eating of more plant base diet which includes more of vegetables, fruits and whole grain. Taking the above listed diet will make you not to worry about alkalinity because it is refers to as healthy diets which eliminate cancers and chronic diseases like hypertension and stroke. Alkaline diets are more vital to kidney health since kidney is easily damage with excess of protein.

Healthy alkaline diets should not eliminate nuts and grains.

WHO CAN TAKE ALKALINE DIET

Alkaline diets are mainly preferred for persons suffering from these health challenges listed below;

- Kidney diseases
- Heart diseases
- Cancer
- Diabetes

Note: you are to tell your health provided for guidance before taking your alkaline diets so as not to harm yourself by cutting out some vital nutrition that might be important to your health.

WHO SHOULD NOT TAKE ALKALINE DIETS

Anybody having traces of preexisting health challenges are not allowed to take alkaline diets. Some persons might not be full when taking alkaline diets unless an addition of protein food.

Some acidic food is needed for a healthy body among which are;

- Eggs
- Walnut

It is notice that the elimination of these acidic food might result in obsessive and inadequate nutrient.

CHAPTER THREE

THE BEST REFLUX- FREE MEAL PLAN THAT CAN SERVE YOU FOR A WEEK

You might be diagnosed of having acid reflux diets or going off the required diet for your healthy living. Persons with acid reflux are tends to avoid certain food that trigger their reflux. Some of these trigger foods are richly high in fat such as tomatoes, caffeine, onion, and chocolate. The one-week diets plan will show you how to avoid reflux diets.

DAY ONE

- **BREAKFAST**: you are to take rice chex cereal with a combination of sliced banana and almond butter.

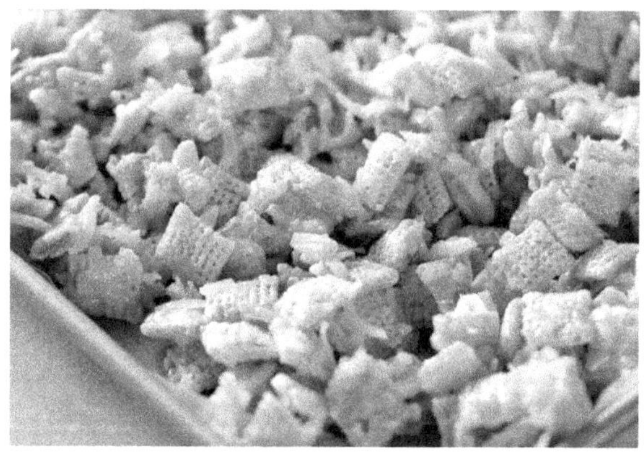

Required Snacks: get an apple, and slice it together with almond milk

- **LUNCH**: Go for a Tuna Salad Wrap.

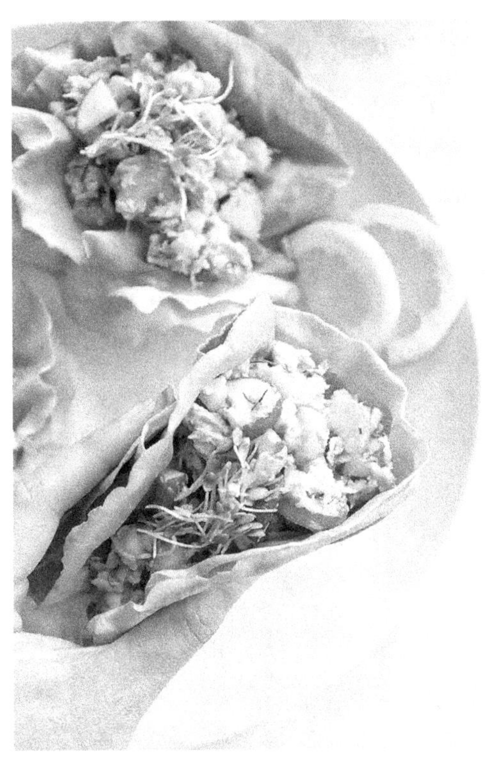

Required   Snacks: prepare banana bar with the use of the following   ingredient;   2   ripe banana, 2 cups of oat flour, 2 eggs, a cup of sugar, baking machine of about 350 degrees until it is ready.

- **DINNER:** Chicken Spaghetti that is Free of Gluten. This is achieved by baking chicken thighs over rice.

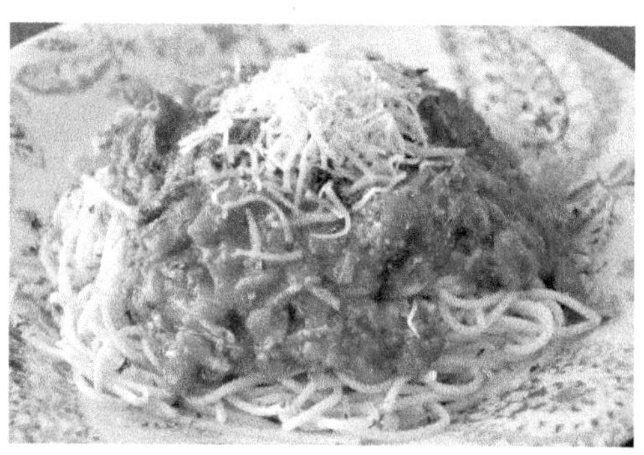

DAY TWO

- **BREAKFAST**: prepare a green smoothie that is from coconut milk, banana, mango and spinach.

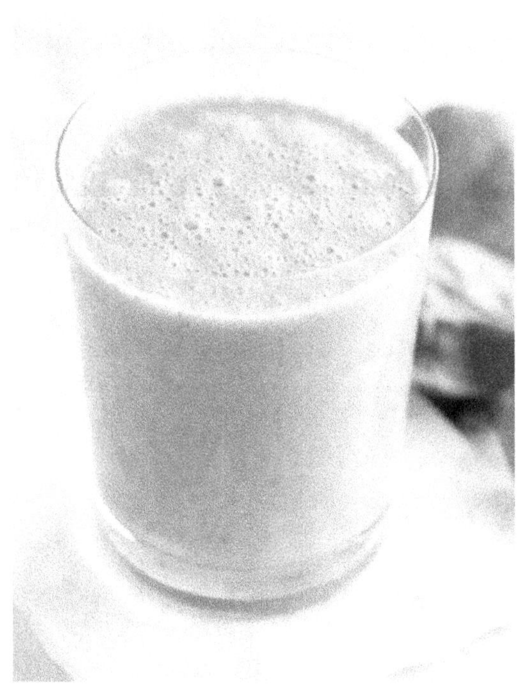

Required snacks: prepare a banana bars as in day one above.

- **LUNCH:** get a peanut butter that is combined with honey sandwich and eating together with a baked potato chip.

Required Snacks: almonds and dates

- **DINNER:** get baked chicken thighs over rice. Prepare it with turkey and avocado wrap.

DAY THREE

- **BREAKFAST:** prepare a nice rice pudding with cooked rice, sugar and rice milk.

Required snacks: Take Granola bar

- **LUNCH:** prepared turkey and avocado wrap

Required snacks: get a baby carrots and hummus

- **DINNER:** prepare a simple homemade shrimp lo-mein that will contain fresh ginger, rice noodles and soy sauce.

Required snacks: Eggs and turkey bacon.

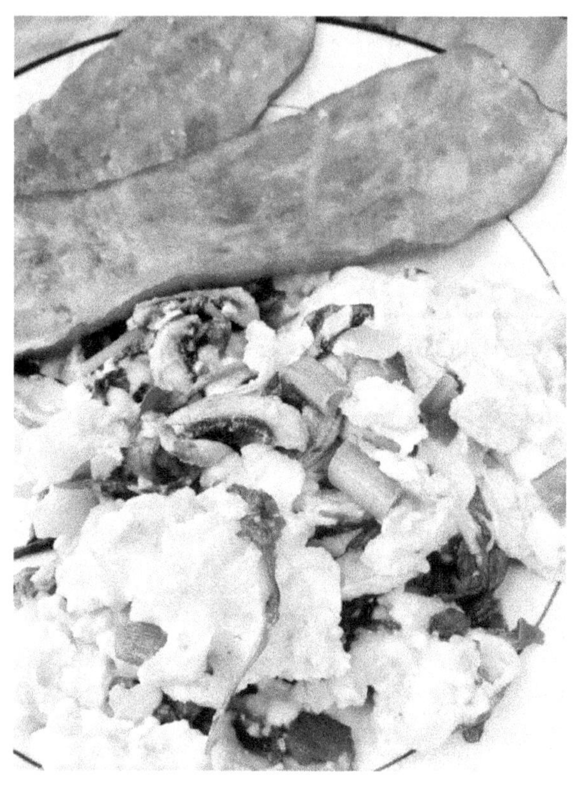

DAY FOUR

- **BREAKFAST:** Eggs and turkey bacon

Required snacks: get a coconut yoghurt with an addition of banana slices

- **LUNCH:** collect some quantity of chicken salad and mixed it up with green topped.

Required snacks: Take the baked rice crackers

- **DINNER:** get some quantity of baked pork chops

Required snacks: get a ZZ and place it over gluten free pasta

DAY FIVE

- **BREAKFAST:** you are expected to take walnuts, oatmeal and maple syrup.

Required snacks: get your desired quantity of rice cakes which should be topped with walnuts butter

- **LUNCH:** get some eggs boiled in combination with crackers and some applesauce

Required snacks: take some popped popcorn

- **DINNER:** get some turkey meatballs with pasta that is free of gluten.

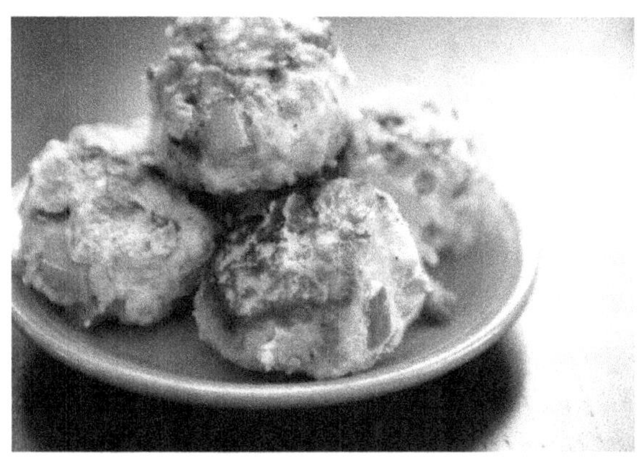

Required snacks: take some rice in combination with honey glazed salmon

DAY SIX

- **BREAKFAST:** prepare a peanut butter smoothie with the following ingredients; banana, milk, peanut butter and yoghurt

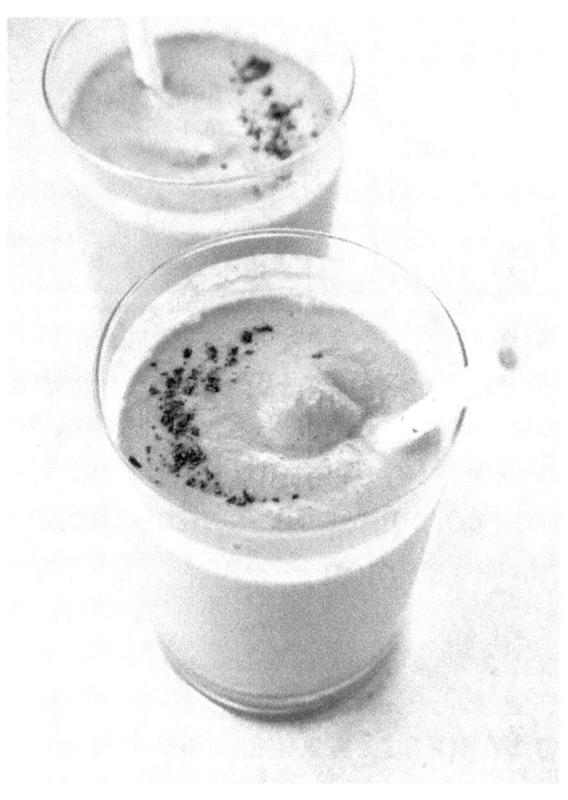

Required snacks: get a trail mix without the addition of chocolate

- **LUNCH:** get some turkey meatballs with pasta that is free of gluten. You are to use mayonnaise in place of tomatoes over the meatballs.

Required snacks: get some quantity of baked potato chip place in a ranch dip

- **DINNER:** get some honey mustard glazed salmon and place it over rice

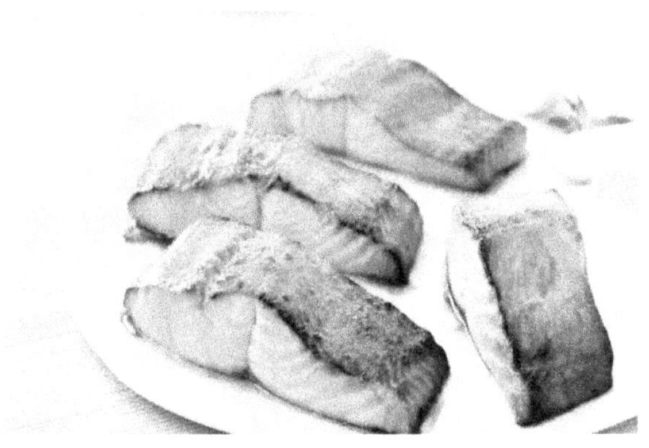

Required snacks: get some slices of apple and add it to peanut butter

DAY SEVEN

- **BREAKFAST:** prepare yoghurt parfait with the following ingredients; banana, Greek yoghurt and blueberries.

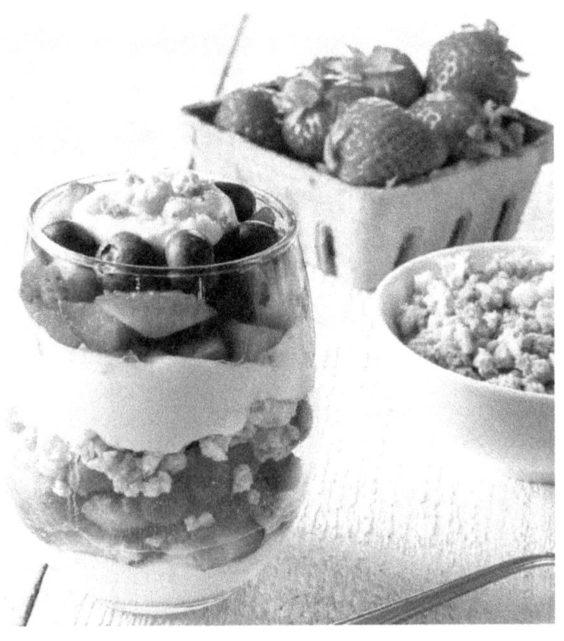

Required snacks: get some slices of apple and add it to peanut butter

- **LUNCH:** get a shrimp salad wrap

Required snacks: get cookies made of Pamela's butter shortbread that is free of gluten.

- **DINNER:** prepare a homemade pizza that is made with the following ingredients; sautéed mushroom, crust that is free of gluten, and melted cheese

CAUSES OF HEARTBURN

It is on record that about 15 million persons suffer from heart burn condition daily in American. There are certain foods and beverages that must be discourage in your daily meal plan so as to reduce heartburn. The timing at which you eat you food and the size of the food must also be put into consideration.

Heartburn is caused as a result of the lower esophageal (LES) sphincter muscle becoming so relax or weaken thereby allowing acids in the stomach to gain easy access into the esophagus.

CHAPTER FOUR

SIMPLIFIED MEAL PLAN THAT HELPS IN PREVENTING HEARTBURN

Below are the steps to follow;

1) Two to three hours after eating any of your daily meal, you are not permitted to lie down. Lying down makes the acid content in the stomach to splash into the LES.

2) You must not eat any item that will weaken or damage the LES muscles. Such item are peppermint, chocolate, alcohol, food, beverages, citrus juice, caffeine, fatty food,

tomatoes, and chili peppers

3) Cultivate the habit of eating little food so that the much food will not splash into the LES. It is better to eat up to five times in little portions than to eat three times in large portions.

4) Try to avoid much fatty food because they normally stay longer in the stomach for it to digest. Fried and greasy food also tend to weaken the LES muscle

5) The LES muscle will be weaken when you take alcohol during or after eating

6) Don't engage yourself in an exercise immediately after eating because it will cause heartburn in many persons. Stay for a duration of 2 hours before exercising yourself if needed

7) It is recommended that you chew gum after eating so as to stimulate saliva production easily. Saliva helps in the neutralization of acidic content in the stomach thereby moving the food content in the stomach directly to the small intestine.

8) Make sure your meal plan do not cause overweight for the body. Overweight will press the stomach

thereby releasing upward pressure into the LES

9) Immediately after eating, you are required to take a small glass of water so as to flush down all the stomach acid that is tending toward the LES

10) Take beverages that are friendly to your heartburn condition. Such beverages are water, noncitrus juices, and mineral water.

11) Eat more of Fiber diet so as to reduce your acid reflux symptoms. Fiber is gotten mainly from unprocessed plant foods such as whole grain, vegetables, nuts, seeds, and fruits.

THE END

www.ingramcontent.com/pod-product-compliance
Lightning Source LLC
Chambersburg PA
CBHW050749250726
48662CB00005B/2107